YOUR KNOWLEDGE HAS VALUE

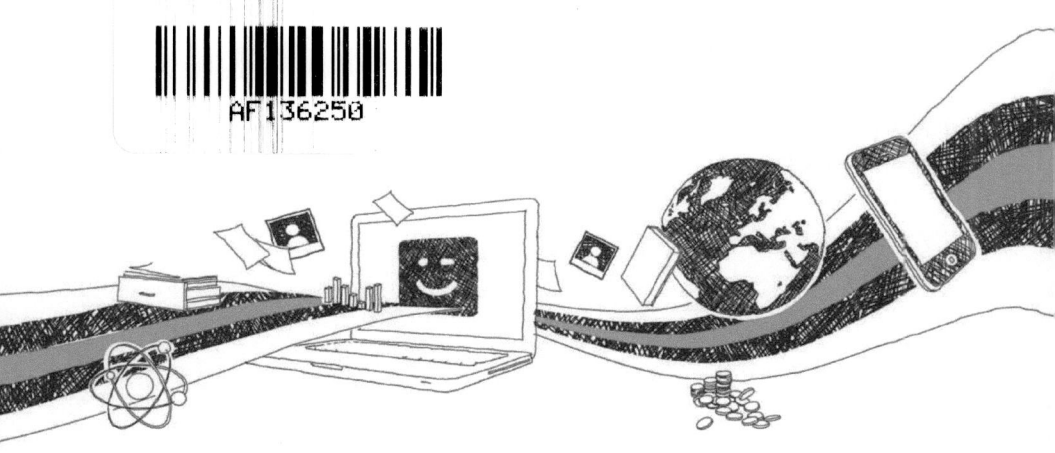
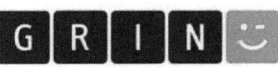

Astha Siwakoti

Weaning among mothers of children in Nepal. Practices, beliefs and taboos

GRIN Publishing

Bibliographic information published by the German National Library:

The German National Library lists this publication in the National Bibliography; detailed bibliographic data are available on the Internet at http://dnb.dnb.de .

Imprint:

Copyright © 2014 GRIN Verlag GmbH
Print and binding: Books on Demand GmbH, Norderstedt Germany
ISBN: 978-3-656-69673-5

This book at GRIN:

http://www.grin.com/en/e-book/276221/weaning-among-mothers-of-children-in-nepal-practices-beliefs-and-taboos

GRIN - Your knowledge has value

Since its foundation in 1998, GRIN has specialized in publishing academic texts by students, college teachers and other academics as e-book and printed book. The website www.grin.com is an ideal platform for presenting term papers, final papers, scientific essays, dissertations and specialist books.

Visit us on the internet:

http://www.grin.com/

http://www.facebook.com/grincom

http://www.twitter.com/grin_com

TITLE OF THE RESEARCH

ASSESSMENT OF PRACTICES, BELIEFS AND TABOOS ON WEANING AMONG
MOTHERS OF CHILDREN IN SINAM VDC OF TAPLEJUNG DISTRICT OF NEPAL

By

Astha siwakoti

For Partial Fulfilment of Masters in Public Health

Rajiv Gandhi University of Health Sciences

Bangalore ,Karnataka

SUMMARY/ABSTRACT

The study was conducted in Sinam VDC of Taplejung district of Nepal. It is descriptive cross sectional study and analysis was done relating independent study variables to dependent variables.

Methods: The data collection methods were used for this study was semi structure questionnaire to assess practice and structured guideline for FGD to understand the beliefs and taboos on weaning in the area.

Results:

A total of 120 mothers with children aged between 3 month to around 3 years were included to assess the weaning practice of which 49.2% were below 1 year, 35% were within 2 years of age, 14.2% less than or of 3 years of age, 1.7% were above 3 years.52.5% of children were male and 47.5% were female.33.3% of families had 2 children and 15.8% of families had 5 children. Majority of them belonged to Janajati(35%) which was predominant ethnic group. Majority of respondents belonged to Hindu religion (66.7%) 34.7% of respondents had primary level of education. There is significant relationship between mother's education and weaning practice in the study. Farming (25%) and foreign employment (51.7%) were major source of income and occupations followed in the area.

90.8% belonged to middle class in the wealth index. Calculations showed that there is positive association between income range and weaning practice.47.5% of mothers introduced weaning foods before 6 months of age of infants, 40% after 6 months and 12.5% before 1 month.
Most common types of weaning foods in this study area were sarbottam pitho(81.8%) and khole (47.1) with rice as a staple diet.85.83% of respondents still breastfed their child along with complementary feeding.14.17% of them expressed their view that breast milk was not sufficient and not required after certain age.75%

of respondents were conscious enough to do night feeding to the baby and remaining 25% were reluctant to the practice.58.3% of respondents had the knowledge on need of sterilization of feeding equipment.72.5% of them had appropriate weaning practice.

Focused group discussion on beliefs and taboos revealed that Cultural factors and taboos have a powerful influence on feeding practices and eating patterns. Young mothers often find it impossible to ignore their ill-informed elders or peer group. Children were being fed three or more meals daily for reasons of hunger and satiety, stomach capacity and adequate growth. Traditional/cultural food preparation beliefs/practices were still adhered to. However, some participants thought that some of these practices were old fashioned and needed to be changed.

Introduction

Child health in developing countries is a serious concern with a large number of children still suffering from malnourishment. South Asian region has the highest global burden of child under nutrition, with almost 41% of children stunted, 16% wasted and 33% underweight. In Nepal the prevalence is 48.3%.[1]

There are various factors that lead to high prevalence of malnutrition in children and among them infant feeding practices is one of the most important. Whether it is breastfeeding or complementary feeding, the practices adopted by mothers or caretakers have direct effect on child health.

World Health Organization (WHO) recommends that children should be exclusively breastfed during the first 6 months of life as breast milk alone is sufficient to meet the nutritional requirements of children till then.[2] In communities undergoing social changes, the incidence and duration of breast-feeding has decreased whereas bottle and solid feeding are introduced earlier.

Complementary feeding is another very important component of infant feeding. After 6 months, mother's milk is not sufficient for the growing child and complementary feeding should be started, timely and in adequate amounts.

Weaning is the process of gradually introducing a mammal infant to what will be its adult diet and withdrawing the supply of its mother's milk.

The process takes place only in mammals, as only mammals produce milk. The infant is considered to be fully weaned once it no longer receives any breast milk (or bottled substitute).[3]

Weaning in human infants is a subject of controversy in terms of its initiation and correct method of doing it. The ideal age of weaning is six months. The desirable weaning food should be inexpensive, home available, clean and easily digestible .It should be rich in calories and protein with adequate amount of trace elements like iron, calcium, vitamins etc.

Weaning is a gradual process starting around the age of 6 months because the mother's milk alone is not sufficient to sustain growth beyond 6 months. Natural weaning occurs as the infant begins to accept increasing amounts and types of complementary feedings while still breastfeeding on demand. When natural weaning is practiced, complete weaning usually takes place between two and four years of age. Planned weaning occurs when the mother decides to wean without receiving signals from the infant that he is ready to stop breastfeeding. It should be supplemented by suitable foods rich in proteins and other nutrients. These are also called supplementary foods. They vary with socio-economic stratification and are regulated by a variety of factors such as education, customs, beliefs and taboos.

Methods

The study design adopted for the study was combination of both quantitative and qualitative study design. The study design was cross sectional, descriptive study. Quantitative methods were applied for assessing the weaning practices and Focused group discussions were done as a part of qualitative study. Focus group discussions were recorded on mobile telephone and interpreted accordingly. The study was conducted for one month (November to December 2013) which included all the study activities for data collection.

Population: Mothers with children aged between 3 months to 3 years in the Sinam VDC of Taplejung district were taken as study population

Sample and sample size: Each VDC consists of 9 wards. The population is not distributed uniformly. All mothers having a child in age group 3 month to 3 year was selected during the study period. According to the previous studies, approximately 70% of mothers have certain beliefs and taboos on weaning. Based on this estimate sample size of 180 mothers was worked out allowing an error of 10% of the estimate.However, 120 mothers were taken as sample that included all mothers of the VDC having infant aged 3 month to 3 years.

Tools and Techniques

Interview was done using Semi structured Questionnaire to assess the weaning practice. Qualitative techniques (FGD) was done to trace out the beliefs and taboos on weaning

Results

Socio demographic variables

Variables	No	Percent
Age group(in months)		
5-15	59	49.2
16-25	42	35
36-45	17	14.2
>45	2	1.7
Sex of infant		
Female	57	47.5
Male	63	52.5
Ethnicity		
Brahmin	32	26.7
Chettri	36	30.0
Janajati	42	35.0
Dalit	10	8.3

Initiation of weaning foods

47.5% of mothers introduced weaning foods before 6 months of age of infants, 40% after 6 months and 12.5% before 1 month.

Initiation of weaning foods

Practice of Breastfeeding	No	Percent
Before 1 month	15	12.5
Before 6 month	57	47.5
After 6 month	48	40
Total	120	100

Appropriateness of weaning practice

It can be inferred that 27.5% of them had inappropriate weaning practice and remaining 72.5% had appropriate weaning practice.

Weaning Practice

Practice of weaning	No	Percent
Inappropriate	33	27.5
Appropriate	87	72.5
Total	120	100

Focus Group Discussion on beliefs and taboos:

Culture has a strong impact on the food behavior of people. The food, habits and practices are closely related to the typical behavior of particular group of people or culture. Such behavior follows codes of conduct in relation to food choice, methods of preparation and eating, number of meals eaten per day, time of eating and size of the portion eaten. Beliefs and practices of breastfeeding and weaning is no exception. It should never be assumed that taboos are just a product of stupidity and ignorance. We need to know more about this absorbing, important and sensitive topic.

Taboos and beliefs on Breastfeeding:

Breastfeeding is the most favored method of feeding newborn infants and children in Nepal. It is almost universal practice during newborn period. Although mothers knew the importance of breastfeeding, the extent of exclusive breastfeeding was less. The practice of giving pre lacteal feeds seemed higher among women of study area. Almost all babies are breastfed. The practice of exclusive breastfeeding wasn't followed. However breastfeeding up to more than recommended six months of age and prolonging it up to 2 to 3 years was reported. Mothers usually started complementary feeding because of their self perception that their breast milk is not sufficient. Majority of mothers breastfed their babies on demand.

Some statements are

'Every pregnant mother does it and I am no exception'

'Breast milk doesn't have any germs'

'Milk is easier to digest to an infant and it's free. We don't have to buy it'

'The baby has no teeth so can't chew other foods'

'My mother breast fed me and so will I to my baby'

'It's a social practice to breastfed and I need to feed something to make baby survive'

Taboos and beliefs on weaning foods: The first weaning food introduced is often a gruel or starchy paste made of maize, rice, oatmeal, wheat, potatoes or crushed plantain (the main ingredient being the local staple) (Brown 1978:2088).Weaning foods in Nepal are based on a staple diet ("dal bhat") of cereal and legume; Locally available ingredients should be used that are low-cost and therefore affordable to the low-income socioeconomic strata. The foods should be soft in texture, low in fiber content, and high in caloric density. In the study area practice of feeding '*khole'* which was prepared from millet or rice was common. The adoption of "sarbottam pitho" (super flour) was preferred from locally available foods by milling beans of different kind, maize ,wheat mixing them in equal proportions. The foods chosen for weaning recipes were easily available from gardens or local markets, low in cost, and used frequently in most households.

Taboos and beliefs on weaning by respondents quoted verbatim are

'It is convenient to feed packed food but it is expensive and cannot afford. It takes lot of time to cook sarbottam pitho. If I had enough money I would change the food items for experimenting. '

'My baby cries without alcohol. My father in law drinks it every 3 or 4 hours. When baby crawls around him, he put drop of it and now it has made him to crave for it. Feeding alcohol is our ritual and pride '

'Giving rice early injures intestine. I feed only liquid and semi solid food '

'Water should be fed soon after birth because they will be thirsty.'

'Our babies are genetically healthy. I feed anything prepared at home from rice, meat, boiled vegetable like pumpkin. They can digest it anyway .Babies of this place

are future military soldiers so we should teach them to eat anything'

'Weather of Taplejung(place) is tonic to all health problems .spices shouldn't be added in food or else anything is healthy'

'Boiled pumpkin should be fed. I change diet observing consistency of stool.'

'I fed biscuit mixed in water because baby used to cry of hunger and preparing gruel food takes time so I opt for noodles soup and biscuit. My baby eats noodles mixed with egg.'

These statements reflect the perceptions and belief systems of respondents or the place as a whole. They considered their babies are genetically healthy and immune because of the weather and diet. Feeding alcohol or letting a baby lick it wasn't considered a bigger behavioral issue. They considered it as a norm and way of teaching cultural practices. Slowly the shift towards feeding commercially packaged food could be possible substitute for traditional home based food.

When asked about their concepts regarding such food-related taboos, mothers considered jaggery as "hot" for the child. Some considered spicy food, papaya, eggs, mangoes etc. "hot" for the child, thus, precluding it from getting these nutritious kinds. Regarding "cold" foods, banana was thought to be "cold" for child by mothers. They considered curd & fruits like guava as "cold foods" for the child. Spicy & fried foods, eggs, tea/coffee, non-vegetarian foods were not considered "harmful" to the child. They had the view that more experimentation with food items should be done to increase the appetite of baby.

Discussion

Systemic efforts had been made to reduce nutrition problems in the country since 1975 by various sectors in Nepal.[4]Few studies have been also conducted to identify nutritional situation in Nepal but studies on child feeding practices especially in complementary feeding were felt lacking since a long time. In this regard, present study was conducted as an attempt to explore more about practices, beliefs and taboos on weaning. A total of 120 mothers with children aged between 3 month to around 3 years were included to assess the weaning practice, appropriateness of behaviour was statistically calculated and associations compared between the study variables. Most of respondents were included who had children below 2 year of age. 52.5% of children were male and 47.5% were female.

Most of the families had 2 child.33.3% of families had 2 children. However, 15.8% of families had 5 children. Parity is one of most influencing factor for weaning practice. 92.1 % of respondents having 1 or 2 children followed appropriate methods of weaning, 75% of them having 2 or 3 children had appropriate practices and only 31% of them with 4 or more children had appropriate practices of weaning. Significant relationship between parity and weaning practice could be inferred from the calculations and chi square value.

A hospital based study in Nepal found almost all (94.82%) mothers fed their infants with only breast milk till the age of one month which came down to 33.19% at the age of 6 months. This evidence shows that the trend of mix feeding is increasing. This phenomenon is true for the developed world as well.[5]

In this study, however 13% of them had initiated weaning before 1 month, 47% before six month and 40% after six month. It was surprising fact that 13% of them actually fed either semi solid or biscuit mixed in water to their infant. Some of them even opted for other items like noodles soup and most commonly cow's milk. Formula milk was not that common because of accessibility and cost issues.

According to the secondary data analysis of Demographic and Health survey of Nepal, 2006 indicated that the rate of introduction of solid, semisolid or soft foods to infants aged 6-8 months was 70%.The study concluded that the complementary feeding rates in Nepal are inadequate except for minimum meal frequency.

However this study showed that only 40% started weaning at correct age (6 month). Most common reason cited in this study, where mothers felt that there was insufficient milk produced and their child was always hungry. Although they were aware about correct timing of weaning, early feeding was seen because they felt the baby would grow faster and cultural belief systems dominated weaning practice.

Most common types of weaning foods in this study area were sarbottam pitho(81.8%)khole (47.1%), and normal family food(69.4%) with rice as a staple diet. Sarbottam pitho is a cereal based flour kind of infant food common in Nepal that is prepared by mixing wheat, maize, soybean, chick peas in relatively equal proportions and grinding it. It is usually cooked in water or cow's milk depending upon taste and availability of milk.

Khole is the local term for infant food comprising of white flour cooked with vegetables or whatever available and adding sugar or salt as preferred by the child..

NDHS reported that more than 35% of mothers gave pre lacteal feeds to their newborns, ranging from 4.3% in Mid Western Hills to 75.7% in Central Terai. There was no difference in this behavior with regards to educational level.

From this study it can be inferred that 27.5% of them had inappropriate weaning practice and remaining 72.5% had appropriate weaning practice. The appropriateness of weaning practice was assessed based on frequency, ingredients and food items fed to the child in a day based on 24 hour recall method.

In a similar study in Nepal about 50% of the mothers fed their child with the food of appropriate consistency and 66.0% fed with the appropriate amount. But only 15.82% mothers fed their children with ideal frequency, sufficient amount and ideal quality.[18]

In this study conduction of focus group discussion revealed a unique kind of perspective towards weaning practice and impact of taboos in it. Nutrition knowledge cannot be the only tool to address the issue. Understanding cultural influences on feeding practices and geographical aspects associated with food habits equally should be integrated in any nutrition intervention to get sustainable impacts.

CONCLUSION

This study was done using both qualitative and quantitative methods of data collection and interpretation. Quantitative methodology was used to address weaning practices among mothers of children in the target group whereas qualitative assessment assisted to analyze the beliefs and taboos prevalent.

The study showed maximum respondents had appropriate weaning practices. It was extremely fascinating to discover that babies in such a rural setting were so healthy and properly fed with nutritious diet. Nutrition education by FCHVs and UNICEF projects played vital role in enhancing the health of infants by using locally available foods.

Focus group interviews in a qualitative research paradigm was effective in exploring and gaining insight into the belief systems and taboos prevalent in the rural setting. Alcohol feeding was a ritual and a belief which respondents quoted as a reason of good health of their children. Blessings of ancestors and genetically strong immune system of people of Taplejung were recorded statements on beliefs of participants that accounted for better health status of children according to them. Hence, these findings might form an important basis for future qualitative studies to explore detailed idea on perceptions and taboos on weaning.

REFERENCES

1) Subba SH, TS chandrashekhar, Binu VS, Joshi HS, Rana MS, Dixit SB-

    Infant feeding practices of mothers in an urban area in Nepal

2) Breastfeeding Guidelines

http://www.wrha.mb.ca/healthinfo/prohealth/files/BF_Guidelines.pdf

(Retrieved 2013-10-28)

3) Wikipedia-https://en.wikipedia.org/wiki/Weaning

(Retrieved 2013-10-30)

4) Nepal Malla Sa and Shrestha SMb: Complementary Feeding Practices and its
Impact on Nutritional Status of under Two Old Children in Urban Areas of the
Kathmandu

5) Ram Hari Chapagain: Complementary Feeding Practices of Nepali Mothers for 6
Months to 24 Months Children

6) Nepal Demographic health survey:

http://www.measuredhs.com/pubs/pdf/SR189/SR189.pdf

(Retrieved 2014-02-17)